DIY Natural Products for Beauty, Health, and Home

Your Ultimate Guide to the Best Natural Home Remedies

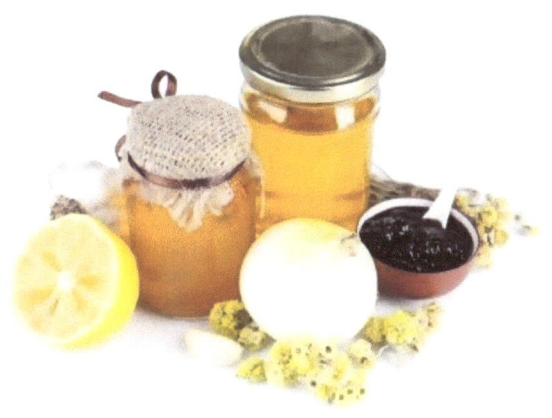

Celeste Jarabese

Table of Contents

Introduction

Gone are the days when concocting your beauty, health and home care products was a teenage girls' slumber party or a woman's only thing! Making your DIY natural products for beauty, home and health is something that you can make it right in your kitchen. Today, so many people are becoming health-savvy and have gained an understanding that the things that we put *on* our bodies affect them as much as what we put *in* them.

In fact, according to research conducted by New York City integrative physician Frank Lipman, over 60% of the products we put on our bodies is absorbed into the bloodstream. Rather than spending too much money on products that you are not so sure of its content; wouldn't it be awesome to make your DIY natural remedies from your kitchen stock? Plus, you won't need to rob a bank to have what you need!

Our kitchens are stocked with natural products such as organic oils, herbs, honey, and apple cider vinegar to name a few. The truth is, you probably have all that you need to make your beauty, health, and home products. You will discover that making your DIY natural products are not just cheaper, but are a healthier alternative compared to the chemicals and preservatives that many companies in the market use today. Plus, it is absolute fun making them.

There are so many upsides for preparing your products at home. You can make some bath salts, facial masks, air fresheners, cleaning agents among other products and package them nicely and give them as gifts to friends and family. You will be amazed at what you can achieve with these simple DIY natural products and how effective household ingredients can be.

Preparing these products will only take you about 20 minutes and cost you less than $20 compared to spending $50-500 on beauty products at the shop. When you take a dollop of coconut oil and mix them up with essential oils of your choice, you can use it to tame skin breakouts, soothe dry skin and even make the perfect lip balm, how cool is that! You may be thinking "I have money, I can afford those products" Well, let me tell you that you aren't just saving on money and time, you are saving your skin as well. Most people react to almost all beauty products released into the market.

Just because a product has been labeled nontoxic does not mean that it is right for your skin. Even as you experiment at home with DIY natural products, it is also important that you understand that not all products might agree with your skin. But the most important thing is that you will feel less pain if you had spent $100 on a product that does not work well with your skin.

It is this kind of sensitive skin that has contributed among many natural enthusiasts to create their natural beauty, health, and home care products. Well, if you are used to expensive synthetic products, the idea of going all DIY natural on your products might sound cliché. However, one thing that I always emphasize is just how simple these products can be. Fresh, natural ingredients have live-enzymes that are often lost during processing, and this is what makes the whole difference for your skin, health, and home. Using natural products are very important to you not just at the cosmetic level, but also at the emotional, mental and spiritual levels. And who among us does not care about a little TLC from time to time? With DIY natural products, you are guaranteed of that extra care with absolutely nothing in exchange- how about that!

CHAPTER 1:
DIY Natural Beauty Products

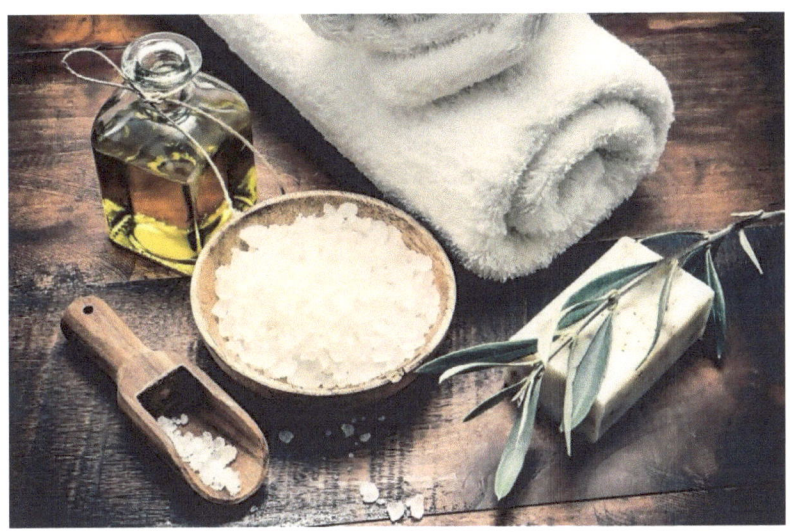

Did you know that cosmetics and beauty products are a major source of exposure to chemicals? According to research, an average beauty product is composed of several harmful chemicals, most of which have not been tested for safety. The good thing is that there are so many natural alternatives that you can use to make your beauty products that will work better on your skin, free of chemicals.

You may be wondering 'but if I have to make natural beauty products for myself, won't I spend so much money on the ingredients?' Well, you are right. You will spend more upfront, but in the long-run, you will not spend a dime. This is mainly because these products are quite versatile and you can use them in various recipes. Like in my case, I only order natural ingredients once or twice a year and am sorted in terms of beauty products for the rest of the year.

For instance, I make a quick natural facial mask using honey. So, all I have to do is to take a warm shower or hold my face over a large bowl of steaming water so that my pores are open. Then I go ahead and apply the warm honey on my face and allow it to sit there for about 20-30 minutes. I then rinse it off with warm water and then splash some cool water to close the pores. Simple and cheap, right? One thing that I love most about honey is that it also works well as a gentle face wash that you can use daily.

The other example I can give is that you can instantly clarify and remove oils from your hair by simply mixing 1 part of white vinegar with five parts distilled water. Then proceed by pouring the mixture onto your hair once you have conditioned. You can add about ten drops of essential oils of your choice; lemon, orange, lavender or peppermint. Also, depending on your hair type, you can detoxify using clay and natural shampoo.

CHAPTER 2:
Common Ingredients for
Natural Beauty Products

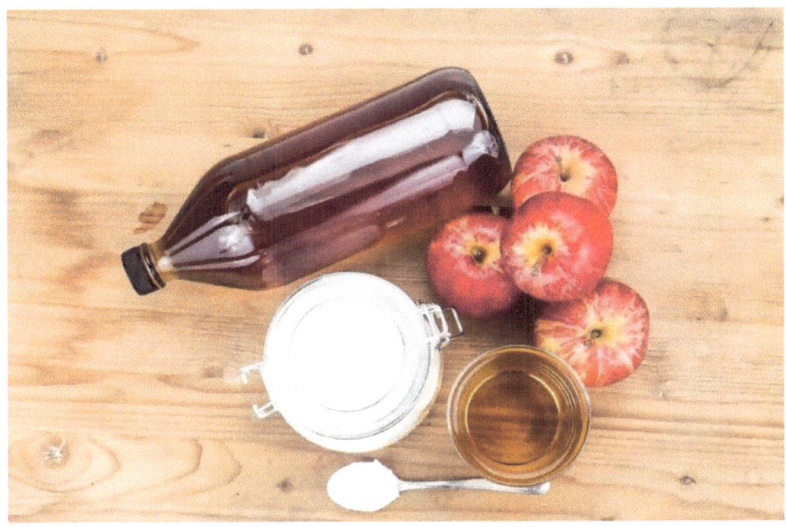

There are so many ingredients that you can use to make your natural beauty products at home. If you are starting with DIY products, these ingredients should be at the top of your list, and you can make as many recipes as you possibly can with just these.

Coconut Oil

Every year, I order about five-gallon buckets of Gold Label Coconut oil from the store. What you need is to get coconut oil that tastes and smells great. The bottom line is to get the best quality coconut oil you can get your hands on, and this is by far the best for me. One thing that you have to realize is that in as much as buying in bulk might cost a lot; the truth is that you save so much. This is because, you can use it to cook, as a skin lotion and when making your natural beauty products. It simply never goes to waste!

If you are sensitive to coconut oil, you can use grass-fed organic beef tallow. However, in as much as it is great on the skin, you will still need to add in some essential oils to mask the mild scent it has. This you can get in a local food store.

Coconut oil has so many skin benefits that include; removing dead skin cells, strengthening underlying epidermal tissues as well as protecting us from sunburns. It also has been shown to have antibacterial, antiviral, antioxidant and antifungal properties. According to research, there is evidence that demonstrates that coconut oil has the potential of fighting skin diseases characterized by such defects on the epidermal barrier function as well as inflammation of the cutaneous tissue.

You can also use coconut oil to make recipes that will help cleanse, remove makeup, moisturize, protect from razor burns as well as healing wounds. As mentioned earlier, coconut oil is also used in cooking, and the good thing with ingesting it is that it offers so many benefits to your looks. In other words, it has healthy fats that nourish your gut and boost the immune system.

Just like any other organ in the body, the skin requires a continuous supply of oxygen and nutrients to remain healthy and flush toxins. Coconut oil is your answer as it helps balance hormonal and digestive functions in the body, hence ensuring optimal skin health.

Tea Tree Oil

Tea tree is scientifically referred to as *Melaleuca alternifolia*. In Australia, tea tree oil has been used for over a century in the treatment of skin breakouts, inflammations, and redness. While so many people tend to react harshly to skin acne treatments, tea tree oil is tolerated and is accompanied by few or no side effects at all.

Just like coconut oil, the tea tree oil is a natural anti-inflammatory, antimicrobial and antifungal ingredient. It is also loaded with rich phytochemicals that make it quite versatile when it comes to skin care. The primary active component of the tea tree oil plays a significant role in reducing harmful bacteria, and this is what makes tea tree oil the best home treatment against acne.

Apple Cider Vinegar

The other versatile and quite inexpensive beauty ingredient is the apple cider vinegar that plays a central role in killing bacteria, cleansing the skin, helping treat acne, antifungal treatment and treating gut issues. The use of apple cider vinegar dates back to 460-377 BC when the Hippocrates mixed it with honey and used the mixture in the treatment of skin sores.

The apple cider vinegar also contains highly beneficial acetic acid as well as important vitamins and minerals like potassium and magnesium. These nutrients play a central role as detoxifying agents especially when they are ingested. It also boosts the liver function and helps balance the bacteria in the gut.

Raw Honey

Since I was a little child, I never missed honey in the kitchen at all. Ever wondered why honey is important when it comes to beauty products? Well, the truth is that raw honey is packed with nutrients, vitamins, enzymes as well as skin-boosting acids. They play a significant role in helping reduce skin breakouts, skin moisturizing, fighting allergies and rashes, healing wounds and scars, as well as containing antiseptic properties. You have to be able to differentiate raw honey from those that have been processed, heated and pasteurized, like those found in the grocery stores. Unlike processed honey, raw honey has its nutrients intact.

Because of its anti-microbial properties, honey is particularly used in dressing wounds and burns. It is also used in the treatment of psoriasis, dandruff, bacterial infections as well as diaper dermatitis. Honey also makes a perfect homemade natural skin care product as a face mask, facial cleanser, and treatment of acne.

Sea Salt

We have seen so many beauty products containing sea salt but have you ever stopped to wonder how you can get your hands on natural sea salt? The good thing with sea salts is that it is loaded with nutrients and minerals such as calcium, magnesium, potassium, and sodium derived from seawater. One interesting thing is that most of these nutrients are similar to the ones found in our skin cells and within our bodies. This is the very reason why real salts play a key role in helping us balance, protect as well as restore the skin to its natural glow.

Some of the best Sea salts that you can use include the Himalayan as well as the Celtic sea salts. They are used in making body scrubs, toners, and facial masks. You can use them with other ingredients that boost the natural glow of your skin such as raw honey, coconut oil, and essential oils. The salt often is reported to have anti-inflammatory properties that soothe the skin and calm skin breakouts, balance skin oil production, help retain skin moisture as well as getting rid of dead skin and irritations.

Therefore, with these benefits and more, you can use the sea salts to make your homemade scrub by simply mixing two teaspoons of seas salt with four teaspoons of raw honey. Then apply this mixture on your skin and rub it around gently and allow it to sit on the skin for about 15 minutes before you can rinse off. You can also use sugar to make your scrub. The good thing with both options is the fact that they are gentle on the skin and you can use it twice a week for a renewal of cells, cell turn-over as well as preventing clogged pores.

Avocado

This is referred to as an ultra-moisturizing fatty fruit that is loaded with vitamins A, D, and E that are absorbed by the skin. This fruit can soothe a sunburned skin while boosting the production of collagen and treatment of age spots and wrinkles. On the other hand, Avocados have anti-inflammatory properties when applied topically as well as when eaten.

To prepare a face mask using an avocado, all you have to do is to whip a fresh avocado with honey, carrier oils and essential oils of your choice. Then apply it on the skin and let it sit for about 20-30 minutes before rinsing it off. The result will be a replenished, well-hydrated skin with a dewy feel.

Lemon Essential Oils

This ingredient has strong antibacterial constituents that play a significant role in lowering the number of dangerous microbial strains, and this explains why it is used as a treatment for acne breakouts. It also is used in fading scars, exfoliating, lightening the skin, toning an oily skin as well as protecting against wrinkling of the skin.

Additionally, the lemon essential oil can be used in making teeth whiteners, laundry fresheners, household cleaners, cellulite creams, and face wash among others DIY natural products for beauty, health, and home use. All you have to do is mix it with Jojoba oil and massage the mixture on parts of your skin that are giving you problems. You can also use the mixture on your hair, and the result is residue-free hair that is shiny and silky.

Argan Oil

This oil is native to Morocco and has been used from generations because of its healing power. It is loaded with high-quality Vitamin A and E, antioxidants, linoleic acid, and omega-6 fatty acids. These nutrients make Argan oil the best when it comes to skin moisturizing as well as boosting the sheen for healthy hair.

You can simply apply a generous amount of Argan oil directly to your skin at least twice a day, and this will soothe skin irritations caused by bug bites, psoriasis, acne, and eczema. The result is skin that feels and looks youthful.

Aloe Vera

If you ask many people about Aloe Vera, the first thing that you will hear is that they use it to heal sunburns. However, what so many of them do not know is that several other benefits come with the use of Aloe Vera. These benefits include; fighting bacteria, soothing skin redness, itching as well as fighting inflammations. For centuries, aloe has been used primarily in the treatment of skin disease, and you can use it as a natural ingredient in preparing your DIY beauty products.

According to recent research results, there is evidence that shows that Aloe Vera is effective in treating wounds and what is even surprising is the fact that it detoxifies the body from the inside out. In other words, when you take Aloe Vera orally, there is a high chance that you will lower the number as well as the size of tumors and parasites present in various body organs like the liver, bone marrow, and spleen.

The thing that makes Aloe Vera very special is the fact that it contains two substances that are used as medicine. These substances include the gel found in the cells at the center of the leaf. The other one is the latex that is derived from Aloe's cells found beneath the skin of the leaves. These substances play a significant role as a natural remedy for frostbites, cold sores, psoriasis, and sunburns.

Biologically, Aloe is considered the most active form of the *Aloe barbadensis miller* species which has over 75 active ingredients such as Vitamins, Fatty acids, lignin, amino acids, anti-inflammatories, enzymes, saccharides as well as salicylic acids. These nutrients are what give the Aloe Vera its anti-microbial and anti-fungal properties, hence making it the number one photodynamic therapy for treatment of the skin.

Jojoba Oil

Did you know that Jojoba oil is the most widely used carrier oil? Well, now you know. This is one of the DIY natural ingredients in beauty products mainly because it is extremely moisturizing and heals a wide range of skin problems that include, psoriasis, acne, wrinkles, scars as well as dermatitis. This ingredient is native to Mexico and the US and has been used as a skin treatment for over a century. It is also used to reduce balding mainly because it boosts hair growth, unclogs the hair follicles and soothes the skin.

The chemical structure of this oil is quite peculiar because it is polyunsaturated wax. Because it is a wax, it makes a perfect skin protectant by providing moisture control and soothing to both the skin and the hair.

Almond Oil

If you are new to using almond oil on your skin, it is high time that you hop onto the beauty bandwagon. This is because almond oil does smell not only amazing but also has antiviral, anti-inflammatory, antiseptic, and antibacterial properties. These properties make it the perfect carrier oil in treating skin rashes, dryness, and acne. You can mix it up with other essential oils when making masks, lotions and homemade body washes that smell great.

Shea Butter

For hundreds of years, Shea butter has been used as a natural skin care product in Africa and across the world. This ingredient makes a perfect moisturizing option for dry skin. It is also pocket-friendly, and hence anyone can afford it and enjoy the benefits it has to offer. These benefits include reducing skin peeling, redness and flaking.

You can simply make your DIY natural skin care butter by mixing it with essential oil of your choices such as eucalyptus, frankincense, lavender oil or bergamot oil to make the perfect lip balm.

Castor Oil

Castor oil is mainly used as drying oil, even though this might seem counterintuitive. You can use it to make DIY natural facial cleanser by taking a small amount like a teaspoon and mixing it with ¼ cup of another oil of your choices such as almond or jojoba oil. Then rub it on your face and massage it. Allow it to sit on the face for about 20-30 minutes and then rinse it off with warm water, hence flushing away skin impurities.

CHAPTER 3:
Natural Skin Care Tips

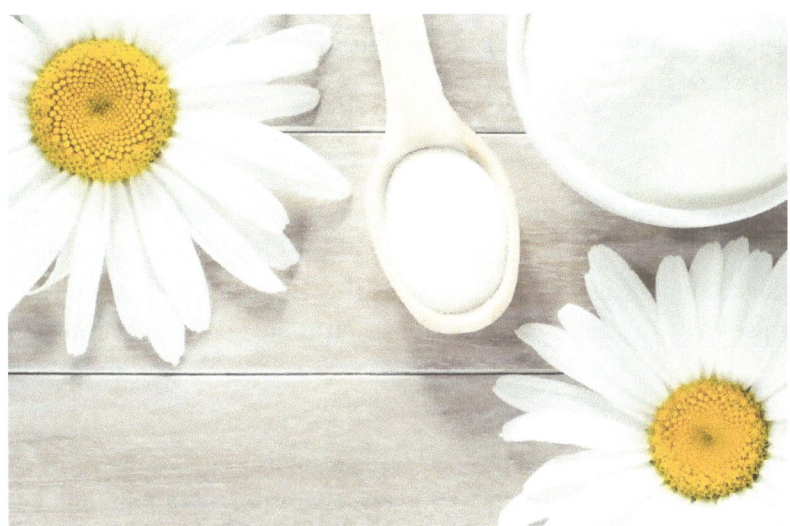

One thing that most people fail to understand is that what we put into our bodies play a big role in what happens on our outer appearance. Yes, the natural ingredients that we have discussed above can be effective in addressing so many skin issues, but you also have to back that up with a healthy diet. If you eat a healthy diet, get good sleep, drink plenty of water and exercise regularly, you can improve your looks tremendously. In addition to these primary lifestyle factors, there are lots of supplements that can help you make the skin more effectively.

In addition to the natural skin care products that we have mentioned above, there are some other products that you can add onto your beauty regimen to help heal the skin, hair and other beauty issues that you might have. Some of these products include;

Probiotics

Over recent years, the benefits of probiotics have moved into the mainstream spotlight, but for a really good reason. The probiotics are simply the good bacteria that help balance the gut microbiome hence boosting the immunity, energy levels, regulation of appetite and control of hormonal balance. In other words, they play a role in helping the immune and nervous system to flush toxins from the body, and this shows up on the skin.

Omega-3 Supplement Cod Liver Oil

Omega-3s are packed with healthy fatty acids the help keep the skin moisturized and elastic. They also play a central role in regulating the hormonal functions, immune functions as well as the nervous system's health. The Cod Liver Oil is also rich in Vitamins A, D, and E as well as omega-3s and antioxidants.

Collagen Protein

This is currently at the top of the list when it comes to natural skin care products. This is mainly because it plays a central role in building healthy skin cells and hence boosting the skin's elasticity, firmness and softness.

In spite of the fact that many beauty products add collagen to boost skin elasticity, the most effective way to have it is to take it internally. The truth is, collagen is a large compound that is not effectively absorbed through the skin, hence making internal ingestion the ideal option for better results.

Drink plenty of water

Ever heard 'water is life,' well that is true. Water is one of the essential things that take good care of your skin and other body organs. According to experts, it is recommended that one takes at least eight glasses of water each day. However, if you suffer from dry skin, taking more would do you so much good. The truth is, water makes up about 70% of the body and a very large portion of the skin as well.

The main aim of taking as much water is to ensure that you flush toxins from the bloodstream and the body cells. In other words, taking plenty of water ensures that you detoxify the body of such things like bacteria and wastes that dull your skin. Without enough water, the skin gets dehydrated, and we appear aged and dull, and the skin becomes a little rough and cracked.

Get plenty of sleep

Did you know that when your stress levels are high, you can barely get enough sleep? Did you also know that these two factors contribute to a hormonal imbalance? Well, the truth is 'beauty sleep' is much more than a saying. Getting enough sleep and lowering your stress levels can go a long way in making magic happen as far as healthy skin is concerned.

When you get enough sleep, you are treating your skin to happy hormones and hence lowering the stress levels. At this point, the body simply has adequate amounts of energy to perform optimal functions such as digestion, repair or worn out skin, regeneration of cells as well as muscle growth. In other words, you simply wake up looking refreshed.

When you do not get adequate sleep, you are exposing the body to similar effects as that caused by stress. This is because, both stress and a lack of sleep make the body conserve energy, hence compromising skin health. Therefore, it is important that you consider implementing natural sleep strategies as a means of busting stress.

Finally, if you suffer from acne among other frequent skin problems, ensure that you are eating a lot of leafy greens. It is also important that you stay away from sugar, gluten, and processed dairy products.

CHAPTER 4
DIY Natural Beauty Products

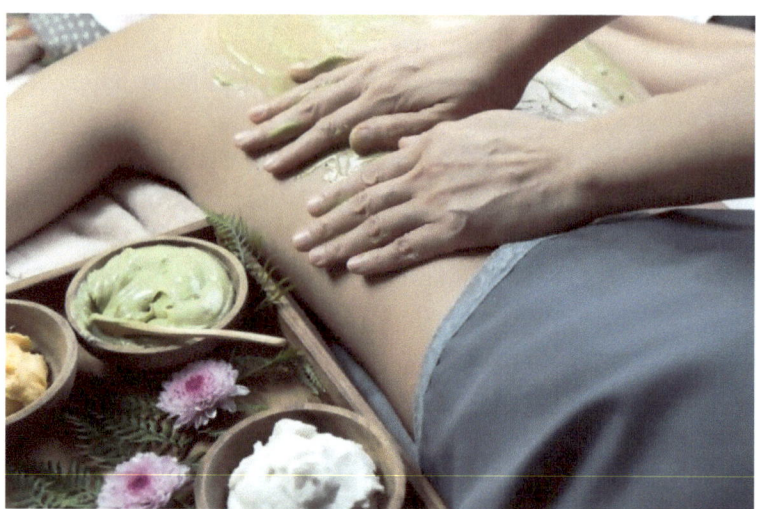

Body Scrubs

Green Tea Scrub

Green tea oil offers many benefits to the skin. The oil has been used to treat itching and a light form of UV protection. It's amazing antioxidant qualities make it an age-defying powerhouse. This body scrub with green tea provides just the right amount of anti-aging oil to green tea balance.

Ingredients

- 1 ½ cup sea salt or organic cane sugar
- ¾ cup of coconut oil
- One tablespoon green tea essential oil
- One teaspoon tea tree oil

Directions

1. Combine ingredients in an airtight jar, mix well and store in a cool place.
2. Moisten skin and scrub with the mixture, wash off.

Hydrating Body Scrub for Baby Soft Skin

This body scrub is full of the goodness of Aloe Vera that works magic by restoring your skin's moisture especially if you have dry skin. It serves as a perfect skin conditioner and is richly loaded with the goodness of vitamin E which nourishes the skin and prevent wrinkling. The most important thing to note is that walnuts are loaded with vitamins and minerals which are good for your skin. Almonds are a good source of vitamin E giving the skin healthy glow. The scrub also serves as a great moisturizer for all skin types because it contains honey.

Ingredients

- One leaf of Aloe Vera
- A handful of walnuts
- A handful of almonds
- Two tablespoons honey

Directions

1. Remove the pulp from the Aloe Vera leaf
2. Grind together all the ingredients to get a coarse paste.
3. Apply the mixture on the skin. Leave it on for 5 minutes. Scrub lightly in circular motions.
4. Wash off with lukewarm water.
5. Always make the scrub fresh and useful. Discard leftovers. This scrub makes the skin soft and supple especially when used at least once a week.

Rice and Honey Whitening Body Scrub

One thing that is important to note about the rice powder is the fact that it has perfect exfoliating properties. It also is important in brightening your skin and making it even toned all through. On the other hand, honey is known to be an organic product that is perfect for moisturizing and soothing your skin while offering it with both antiaging and antibacterial properties. A combination of rice and honey makes an incredible body scrub that not only leaves your skin glowing, but also makes it supple and soft.

Ingredients

- 6 tablespoons honey
- 2 ½ cups rice, ground to a coarse texture
- 15-20 drops almond oil (use only for dry skin)

Directions

1. Start by combining all your ingredients in an airtight container and then close it and shake it to mix. Ensure that they are mixed very well to achieve a uniform consistency.
2. Then store it in a cool dry place.
3. To use, simply moisten your skin with water and then apply a generous amount of the scrub on your body
4. Gently massage the scrub on your skin and let it sit for a couple of minutes before washing it off.

Summer Red Lentil Body Scrub

This body scrub is made from Rose water which plays a significant role in making you feel refreshed especially during the summer. It also offers relieve for itchiness or burning sensations on the skin.

This body scrub also boasts of the goodness of honey which is a great moisturizer that is loaded with antibacterial and anti-oxidant properties. It is also suitable for use by all skin types and leaves the skin supple. On the other hand, the red lentils come in to get rid of dead cells leaving your skin with a healthy glow.

Ingredients

- 1 ½ cup red lentils, ground to a coarse texture
- 5 tablespoons rose water
- 7 tablespoons honey

Directions

1. Simply combine all these ingredients in a sterile airtight container.
2. Close it and shake well to mix until the mixture is uniform
3. Store in a cool dry place
4. To use, simply take a generous portion and apply it on a moistened skin and scrub gently
5. Allow it to sit on the skin for a couple of minutes and then thoroughly rinse it off with clean cold or lukewarm water.

Red Lentil Body Scrub for Winter

Did you know that winter can strip your skin of its natural moisture? Well, if you have a dry skin, then trust me, normal moisturizing during winter will not help one bit. This is where your organic ghee comes in to rescue the situation.

Organic ghee serves as a great natural skin moisturizer and it works wonders especially when used on dry skin leaving it soft and supple. The added red lentils go a long way in helping get rid of dead cells from the skin leaving you with a healthy glow.

Ingredients
- 1 cup ghee
- 2 ½ cup red lentils, ground to a coarse texture
- Rose essential oil (to neutralize the strong aroma of ghee)

Directions
1. Start by combining all your ingredients in a sterile airtight container
2. Close the jar and shake it to mix well until the consistency is even
3. Store your scrub in a cool, dry place.
4. To use, start by moistening your skin with water and then apply a generous amount of scrub all over your body and gently massage it.
5. Wash off with plenty of clean water

Body Lotion

Ultra-Moisturizing Lotion

Shea butter is one of the products that is loaded with skin moisturizing properties. It acts by reducing wrinkles on the skin. It also is great in the treatment of eczema and other similar skin conditions. This lotion also contains tea tree oil which has anti-bacterial properties that help fight pimples and maintain a blemish-free skin. The essential oils help to soothe the skin and also relax the senses. It also contains almond oil which is rich in vitamin E, hence making it the perfect elixir for younger looking skin.

Ingredients

- 1 cup Shea butter
- Four tablespoons avocado oil or sweet almond oil or jojoba oil
- 30 drops lavender essential oil
- 20 drops rosemary essential oil
- 15 drops carrot seed oil
- 10 drops tea tree oil

Directions

1. Place a saucepan over medium-low heat. Add in Shea butter and the essential oil that you like based on your taste and preference. When it is melted, remove from heat. Transfer into a bowl.
2. Place the bowl in the freezer to cool for about 15-20 minutes until it is slightly solid.
3. Add lavender oil, rosemary oil, carrot seed oil, and tea tree oil. Whisk until the mixture is creamy. (You can do this manually or if you want you can use the whisk attachment of your mixer)
4. Spoon into a clean and dry jar. Keep it in a dry and cool place at room temperature.
5. Apply a small amount on the body as well as face whenever required.

Nourishing Rose and Almond Moisturizer

Cocoa butter, Shea Butter, and coconut oil are great natural skin moisturizers that help you maintain soft and supple skin. Almond oil helps to nourish the skin from within and has reduces fine lines and wrinkles.

Ingredients

- ½ cup of coconut oil
- ¼ cup Shea butter
- ¼ cup of cocoa butter
- Two tablespoons rose water
- Two tablespoons almond oil
- Ten drops rose essential oil

Directions

1. Add Shea butter, coconut oil, and coconut butter to a saucepan. Place the pan over low heat. When all ingredients are melted, remove mixture from heat.
2. Add rose, almond oil, and rose essential oil. Whisk thoroughly until you get the desired texture.
3. Transfer into an airtight container and keep this moisturizer in a cool, dry place.

Double Chocolate Lotion

One thing that I love about this lotion is its divine scent. Once you are done washing your hands, apply this lotion to slow down aging on your hands and feet.

Ingredients
- 2 teaspoons cocoa essential oil
- 3 cups pure distilled water
- 2 cups cocoa butter
- 1 cup jojoba oil
- 1 cup grated beeswax
- 3 ½ teaspoons Vitamin E oil

Directions
1. Start by placing all your ingredients in a saucepan and then heat it on low heat.
2. When the ingredients begin to melt down, gently mix them together and remove the saucepan and let it sit for about 10 minutes.
3. Once the lotion is cool enough, pour it into a sterile airtight container and keep it in a cool dry place.
4. To use, simply take a generous amount and rub it on your hands and legs and massage gently.

Raspberry Almond lotion

Did you know that raspberry seed oil serves as an antioxidant powerhouse? It is loaded with the goodness of both Omega-3 and Omega-6 oils. Do not confuse raspberry seed oil and raspberry oil because these two are very different from each other.

Ingredients

- 1 cup almond oil
- 3 cups grated beeswax
- 5 teaspoons raspberry seed oil
- 1 teaspoon vitamin E oil
- ¾ cup pure Aloe Vera gel

Directions

1. Start by placing all your ingredients in a saucepan and then allowing it to cook on low heat until all of them melt and come together.
2. Mix it together to achieve a uniform consistency and let it sit at room temperature for about 15 minutes
3. Pour your lotion into a sterile airtight container and store it in a cool dry place
4. To use, simply dispense a generous amount onto your hands and apply it onto your body while massaging gently.

Grapefruit Zing Lotion

This is the best lotion to say "good morning" to your beautiful skin. This is because the scent is not only amazing but also is packed with the goodness of essential oils that go a long way in helping your skin get rid of pimples leaving it smooth and flawless.

Ingredients
- 1 cup grated beeswax
- 2 teaspoons Vitamin E oil
- 4 teaspoons grapefruit essential oil
- 2 ½ cups coconut oil
- 1 cup pure Aloe Vera Gel

Directions
1. Start by placing all your ingredients in a saucepan and let it heat under low heat while constantly mixing until everything melts and comes together
2. Turn off the heat and let the mixture stand for about 10 minutes
3. Pour your lotion into a sterile airtight container
4. To use, dispense a generous amount onto your hands and massage it onto your body and enjoy the scent and all the benefits it comes packed in it.

Body Buttercreams

Anti-Aging Face Cream

Shea butter restores the skin moisture. Rose water rejuvenates the skin. This anti-aging butter cream plays a central role in helping your skin retain moisture hence fighting signs of aging. Wheat germ tightens skin cells and improves its elasticity.

Ingredients

- Eight teaspoons beeswax, grated
- Four tablespoons rosewater
- ¼ cup Shea butter
- Eight teaspoons wheat germ oil
- Four tablespoons sweet almond oil
- Four teaspoons organic honey
- 10 drops carrot seed oil
- Ten drops rose oil or any essential oil of your choice

Directions

1. Place the beeswax in a glass container and then on a double boiler under low heat.
2. Pour the rosewater in a cup and place the cup in the double boiler along with the beeswax. Similarly, warm the honey.
3. When beeswax is melted, add Shea butter and constantly stir until it melts and is well blended.
4. Add wheat germ oil and sweet almond oil. Using an immersion blender or hand mixer, whip the mixture together until they are well blended. Add the warmed rose water and honey slowly, whipping simultaneously.
5. Remove from the heat. Stir constantly until it is cooled.
6. Add essential oils. Stir well.
7. Scoop it into a glass jar. Cover tightly with a lid.

Hawaiian Body Butter

Slather this amazing body butter scented on your skin to reap the benefits of pineapple and mango. This butter is loaded with mango and pineapple goodness which makes it perfect for anti-aging. It also has the ability to reduce those irritating wrinkle lines that begin to appear as you age. It also contains coconut oil and Vitamin E which helps leave your skin feeling soft and lovely.

Ingredients

- One teaspoon pineapple essential oil
- ½ cup mango butter
- 1 cup of coconut oil
- One teaspoon vitamin E oil

Directions

1. Place ingredients in a glass bowl and beat until smooth.
2. Scoop the butter into a sterile airtight jars and store it in a cool, dry place.

Cinnamon Body Butter

What draws me to this body cream is the comfy scent of cinnamon that makes you feel at home. Cinnamon is packed with antibacterial properties making it wonderful for use on the skin. It leaves both the skin and the joints feeling smooth and supple while offering it a soothing feel.

Ingredients

- 3 ½ cups cocoa butter
- 4 teaspoons cinnamon essential oil
- 1 cup Argan oil
- 5 teaspoons Arabica seed oil

Directions

1. Start by putting water into the saucepan so that is it halfway filled
2. Bring the water to heat over medium heat
3. Now, in a glass bowl, add your cocoa butter and coconut oil and allow it to melt
4. Then remove it and set aside to cool
5. Into the mixture, add in all the remaining ingredients and stir well to achieve a uniform consistency
6. Allow the mixture to cool in a refrigerator for about 30 minutes
7. Now, use a hand immersion blender to beat the butter cream together and then scoop and put it in a sterile airtight container.
8. Store in a cool dry place

Citrus Body Butter for Glowing skin

The tea tree oil in this body butter offer fantastic anti-bacterial properties while the orange essential oil gives you that fresh scent that keeps your mind alert. The extra virgin coconut oil and the Shea butter are good moisturizers and keeps your skin soft and supple throughout the day.

Ingredients

- 15 drops lemon essential oil
- 25 drops sweet orange essential oil
- 5 drops tea tree oil
- 3 cups extra virgin coconut Oil
- 10.5 ounces Shea Butter

Directions

1. Start by mixing the coconut oil and Shea butter in a large Mason jar and cover it tightly.
2. Now, create a water bath in a saucepan and the mixture in your Mason jar into the saucepan with water and allow the mixture to melt.
3. Once the ingredients have melted, remove the mixture from the heat and add in the tea tree oil and the other essential oils.
4. Mix them together and allow it to cool at room temperature for about half an hour.
5. Then place the mixture in the freezer for about 10 minutes or until the butter is completely solidified.
6. Remove it from the freezer and start whipping it together using a whisk until it achieves a uniform consistency.
7. Soon the butter into a sterile airtight container and store it in a cool dry place.

Vanilla Bean Body Butter

This is the body butter that will rejuvenate your skin and leave you feeling relaxed throughout the day, thanks to it soothing aroma of vanilla. It is very pleasant and goes a long way in giving you a relaxed mind and body. It is packed with coca butter that deeply nourishes the skin. The almond oil on the other hand is loaded with Vitamin E oil that give your skin a youthful healthy glow.

Ingredients

- 3 ½ vanilla bean pods
- 1 cup sweet almond oil
- ¾ cup coconut oil
- 3 cups raw cocoa butter

Directions

1. In a small pan, add in your coconut oil and cocoa butter and bring it to melt under low heat
2. Once all the ingredients are properly melted, turn off the heat and set the pan aside to cool at room temperature
3. Now, using a food processor, grind the vanilla beans
4. Add the ground vanilla beans and sweet almond oil into the cooled mixture of coconut oil and cocoa butter.
5. Stir to mix well and freeze it for about half-an hour.

CHAPTER 5:
DIY Natural Products
for Your Home

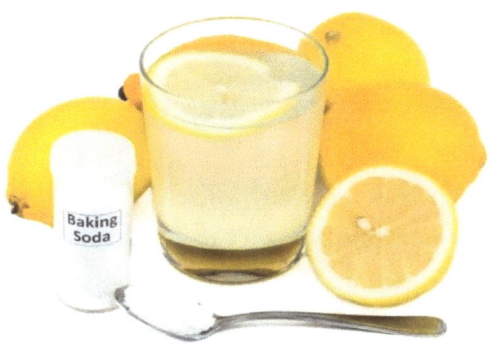

For so many years, I have been using DIY natural products for cleaning my home and have never looked back. For me, initially, this was all about saving money considering that the cost of cleaning products is high. However, with time, I started seeing the benefits of using natural home products for cleaning because they worked and did not have any side effects. Some of my family have very sensitive skin because most of the store-bought products contain chemicals that are irritating to the eyes and the skin. Using natural products for home cleaning has been a plus for us, and hence the reason why over the years I have replaced commercial products for homemade versions.

Did you know that there are natural solutions to almost every cleaning task you have at home? Well, the truth is, indeed there are so many natural products that you have in the kitchen that make perfect cleaning agents. Some of the natural DIY cleaning products that you can include:

- All-purpose cleaners
- Reusable antimicrobial wipes

- Floor cleaners
- Linen cupboard Deodorant
- Fridge cleaners

Trust me, making your homemade cleaning products is super easy. You will be surprised that you have these ingredients already in your kitchen. Some of my favorite ingredients for making natural cleaning products include:

Baking Soda

This is also referred to as *bicarbonate powder*. It is indeed an ideal deodorizer when you are looking for something to get rid of bad smells in the house. It also doubles up as an effective antiviral agent that plays a central role in eliminating grime and grease on surfaces especially when it is used together with vinegar. You can simply use the baking soda that you can find on your baking aisle.

White Vinegar

White vinegar has natural acidity that makes it the perfect anti-bacterial and anti-fungal disinfectant that can cut through grease, descale and also serve as a great glass cleaner. There are so many ways in which you can use white vinegar for cleaning, and you can easily find them sold at the grocery store. My favorite is the one from home brand but you can always find a variety on the dressing isle at the supermarket.

Essential Oils

One thing that I love about essential oils is the fact that they make the perfect air fresheners by giving your product a pleasant smell. However, what you have to appreciate is that other benefits come along with using essential oils in your home cleaners other than giving your home a nice smell. Lavender and tea tree oil in natural cleaning products serve as antibacterial agents and disinfects surfaces in your home. Some of the best essential oils that you can use include; Eucalyptus, wild orange, lemon, lavender, and tea tree oils.

Detergents

The best detergents that you can use are those that have a neutral pH, are free of fragrance and are septic tank safe. These detergents are very effective in lifting dirt, cutting through grease and grime. These are usually available at a local supermarket as well as eco-stores around you.

Salt

The standard here is the normal table salt that you use in the kitchen. Salt is very effective as a scouring agent. The best thing that you can do is to pour salt on a bowl and mix it with hot water and then pour it down the kitchen sink regularly to ward off foul smells and cut through grease and prevent it from building up. You can also add lemon essential oils and use the mixture to get rid of stubborn coffee and tea stains in cups. If you add baking soda and white vinegar, you get the perfect abrasive cleaner.

Borax

Powdered borax is white and has soft colorless crystals that can easily dissolve in water. You can get borax at the supermarket. So many people wonder whether borax is natural. Well, I have tried doing lots of research on this, and I cannot find anything that proves that it is not natural. My opinion is that it is safe when I use it in my cleaning products. It is very effective in cleaning just about everything in my home.

When cleaning, you need a cloth and spray bottle. The best cloth when it comes to cleaning is the micro-fiber ones since they are reusable. All you have to do is to throw them into the wash and hang them out to dry. For wiping grease, toilets and pet puddles, paper towels come in handy. On the other hand, when you make homemade cleaners, it is important that you have a spray bottle. You can get a wide variety of spray bottles at the grocery store near you. Some people say that glass bottles are better especially when using essential oils. However, my preference has always been plastic since I knock my bottles during cleaner and with plastic, I don't have to worry too much about breaking, plus, they are pocket-friendly compared to glass.

CHAPTER 6:
Natural Home Cleaning Products

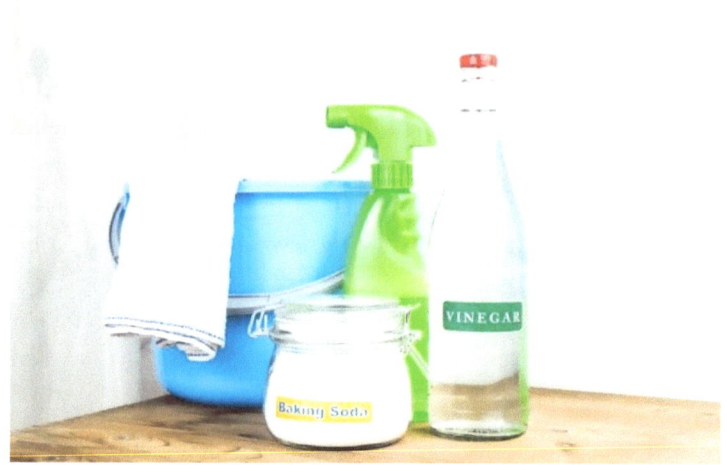

All-Purpose Cleaner

One of the widely-used cleaning agents is white vinegar. It is very useful if you want to keep your home clean and free of mold. Baking soda together with white vinegar make a great all-purpose cleaner. Simply add a few drops of tea tree or lemon essential oils to enhance its ability to disinfect surfaces.

What you need to make an all-purpose cleaner:

- ½ cup white vinegar
- 2 tablespoons baking soda
- 10-15 drops of tea tree essential oil or lemon essential oil

Directions
The first thing is to combine white vinegar with essential oils of your choice in a spray bottle. Then add to it baking soda and mix thoroughly. Pour enough water

to fill the bottle and shake well to ensure that all ingredients are properly mixed. Once it is ready for use, simply spray the area that you would like to clean and use a cloth to wipe it clean.

Tile Cleaner

One thing that I have come to realize is that the commercial tile cleaners that are sold at the supermarket or home stores are filled with lots of contaminants. In fact, according to research, most of these chemicals have been linked with damage to the reproductive system, hormonal imbalances as well as being cancer agents. An analysis conducted in 2009 reported that benzene, formaldehyde, and toluene, which are components of gasoline, are found in most tile cleaners.

Well, the good news is that you can get rid of them and make your eco-friendly tile cleaner that is free of chemicals. To make the tile cleaner, you need:

- A cup baking soda
- Liquid castile soap
- Fifteen drops of essential oils. I mostly use lavender or tea tree essential oils for my tile cleaner.

Directions

All you need is to place the baking soda in a large mixing bowl and then slowly pour in the castile soap while stirring until it looks like frosting. Add to the mixture the essential oil of your choice. To use, you need a sponge which you then dip into the mixture and use it to scrub the tiles thoroughly. Rinse the tiles with clean water. To add more power to it, you can cut a lemon in half and use in place of a sponge.

Disinfectant Wipes

Here, you can use vinegar as your primary ingredient in making disinfectant wipes. You can also add in essential oils such as lemon, eucalyptus or tea tree to give it more power. To prepare this, you need:

- 2 cups of water
- ½ cup white vinegar
- 15 drops each of tea tree, eucalyptus and lemon essential oils
- An empty container such as an old baby wipe container
- 20 squares of cloth (You can make this from an old T-shirt, dish towel or even any other similar material that is available to you)

Direction

The first step is for you to obtain clean clothes that you have folded into squares. Then place them in an empty container and set that aside. Now, in a large bowl, combine water, your white vinegar, and all three essential oils and stir until they are mixed well. Pour the mixture into the container with your wipe cloths. Allow them to soak the solution for a couple of minutes. When you are ready to use, pull out and use just like you would a store-bought wipe.

Glass Cleaner

Most of the commercial glass cleaners that we get from the store often are irritating and aggravate allergies and asthma among other health reactions associated with its use. However, despite these side effects, it does a fabulous job. This is mainly because it contains an orange essential oil that is derived from orange peels. This orange oil is loaded with a d-limonene compound that makes one of the best cleaning agents, especially for glass.

To prepare this, you will need:

- ½ cup white vinegar
- ½ teaspoon natural liquid dish soap
- 3 cups of water
- 15 drops of orange essential oil

Directions

The first thing is to put all your ingredients in a spray bottle and then shake very well to mix. When you are ready to use it, simply spray it directly onto the glass surface to be cleaner and then wipe it off. If the spots on your glass surface are tough, use a rough kitchen sponge to scrub it off and then repeat by spraying and wiping it clean. If there are liquids that collect at the bottom of the window pane, the best thing that you can do is to use a cotton cloth to wipe it off.

All-Purpose Bathroom Cleaner

The bathroom is often one of the toughest rooms in the house to clean. This means that, if you are going to clean it to achieve a sparkle, you need powerful bathroom cleaners to do the job. This recipe is absolutely what you need to get rid of those tough stains. Ever heard of washing soda? Well, this is what you need to get the job done.

Washing soda simply refers to the sodium salt of carbonic acid that is soluble in water. The fact that it has proportions of carbon, sodium, and hydrogen, it makes it quite an effective cleaning booster. You can find it in the laundry section at your local grocery store. You can also get them to build online among other places that sell cleaning agents.

The good thing is that you can make yours pretty easily. Here are the things you need:

- 1 ½ teaspoons Borax
- 1 ½ teaspoons washing soda
- 1 ½ teaspoons castile soap (liquid form)
- 2 ½ cups of boiling water
- ¾ cup white vinegar
- Twenty drops of essential oils; you can use tea tree, eucalyptus, lemon, and grapefruit essential oils.

Direction

In a large mixing bowl, simply combine the Borax, washing soda, white vinegar, and castile soap. Gradually add in water and stir until all the solutes are dissolved. Allow the mixture to sit for a while until it is cool and then add in your essential oils. Pour the mixture into a 24 oz. Spray bottle and shake well to mix. You can use a funnel to pour the mixture into the spray bottle to avoid losing the solution.

To prepare your washing soda, you need baking soda, an oven, and a large dish. Start by pre-heating your oven to 400° Fahrenheit. Then pour about an inch-thick layer of baking soda onto the bottom of a baking dish. Place it in the oven for like an hour with stirring at least once or twice during the process. Once it is ready, it should have changed from a powder feel to grainy feel. Let it cool before you can transfer it into an airtight jar.

Tub and Shower Cleaner

You thought the bathroom was the toughest to clean? Well, the shower and the tub are much more than that! This means that you will need even more powerful cleaners to get the job done. This recipe works the magic, and it is easy to prepare and use in erasing tough stains, hard water deposits, and soap scums without necessarily leaving you feeling as though you just went through a marathon. Well, you may be a little skeptical at how simple this is, but trust me, it works the magic!

You simply need:

1-part vinegar and 1-part natural dishwashing soap and a spray bottle. Simply measure equal parts of these two ingredients such that, if you are using two cups of vinegar, you will need two cups of natural dishwashing soap as well. Put the vinegar in a large bowl and place it in the microwave and heat until it is hot. Pour the vinegar into a sterile spray bottle. Add in the dish washing soap and shake thoroughly until they are uniformly mixed.

To use it, simply ensure that the bathroom is well ventilated by turning on the fan and opening all windows because the solution has a strong vinegar smell. Then spray a generous amount of the mixture onto the shower and tub and allow it to sit for about 30-45 minutes. After that, scrub it thoroughly using a sponge and brush and then rinse off with clean water.

Dusting Solution

Dust often accumulates in the house quite easy and is loaded with harmful compounds such as flame retardants, pesticides and other harmful chemicals in the air. Well, you may be thinking, 'but I have a dust cleaner that can do the job' the truth is, most of the store-bought dust cleaners are packed with even more harmful contaminants along them hormone-disrupting chemicals. With this dusting solution that is easy to mix on your own, you can dust all the surfaces in the house.

To prepare this duct cleaner, you'll need:

- Three tablespoons of 100% pure lemon juice
- Ten-fifteen drops of extra virgin olive oil
- Ten-fifteen drops of lemon essential oil

Directions

To prepare the dust cleaner, all you need is to add all the ingredients into a spray bottle and shake well to mix. Then spray the mixture directly onto dusty surfaces and use a cotton cloth to wipe off the dust. Store it in a cool, dry place and ensure that you shake well before use.

Carpet Stain Remover

To remove stubborn carpet stains, you need the following to prepare a homemade carpet stain remover;

Enough baking soda to cover the stain.

- 3 cups of warm water
- 1 ½ tablespoons white vinegar
- 1 ½ tablespoons natural liquid dishwashing soap

Direction

Sprinkle the stain with sufficient amounts of baking soda. Then allow this to sit for about 15 minutes before you can vacuum it up. Then combine the natural dishwashing soap, water, and white vinegar in a large bowl and mix well. Sponge the mixture and rub it on the stain and blot using a dry cloth. Repeat this as many times as you possibly can until the stain disappears.

Chapter 7:
DIY Natural Health Products

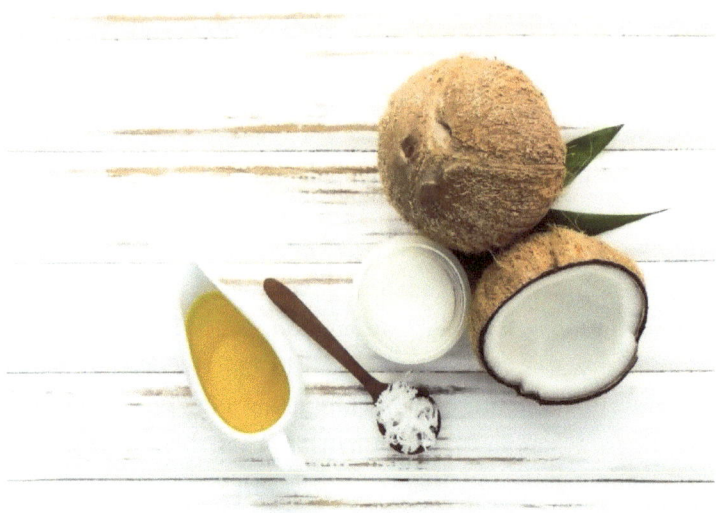

There is a wide range of natural products that play a significant role in helping us make homemade health products that value to our bodies. So many researches have been done to study plant energetics and their mechanisms of actions. What is interesting is the fact that there are so many of these herbs that we can use to make natural homemade remedies that alleviate allergies, skin dryness, irritations, wounds and headaches among other health issues.

Here are some DIY healing salves that you can use to alleviate a wide range of common health concerns at home:

Healing Salve for Allergies

Seasonal allergies are a common condition with symptoms that include wheezing, running noses, stuffy noses, itchy eyes, and more. While seasonal allergies are generally harmless and not life-threatening, they can be a serious irritation. So much so, that most people who suffer seasonal allergies seek herbal relief.

Seasonal allergies can be treated using traditional remedies that include over-the-counter medications. This salve can be used as a vapor rub which is applied to the chest and upper neck three times a day. It contains a lemon essential oil which is photo-sensitive and hence requires you to store it in a dark bottle and away from direct sunlight.

To prepare this salve, you will need:

- One fl. oz. of Castor Oil (2 Tbsp., 30ml)
- Eight fl. oz. of Coconut Oil, 100% Pure, Virgin, Unrefined (16 US Tbsp., 1 cup, 240ml)
- Four fl. oz. of Extra Virgin Olive Oil (8 Tbsp., ½ cup, 120ml)
- 1000 IU of squeezed Vitamin E Oil from a capsule (optional)
- 25-30 drops each of such essential oils such as Basil which has antibacterial properties, Eucalyptus known to treats sinus and respiratory concerns, Lemon which treats respiratory concerns, Peppermint which reduces inflammation, and Tea Tree with antiseptic properties and is known to treat rashes.

Directions

1. Soften the coconut oil by placing it in a bowl of hot water ensuring that the water level should be no higher than half the container with the coconut oil.
2. Measure out the required amount of coconut oil into your 16 oz — Mason jar.
3. Next, add the essential oils, any other carrier oils, and Vitamin E Oil to the coconut oil in the 16 oz. Mason jar.

4. Stir the oils into the coconut oil with stir sticks, stainless steel or wooden spoon.
5. Label your salve with the key essential oils, one use for the salve, and the date you made the salve.
6. Put a lid on the Mason jar and store at a temperature below 76 degrees (24 Celsius) to solidify.

Healing Salve for Arthritis

Some of the signs that one has arthritis include pain, swelling, stiffness and a stunted range of motion. It is important that you seek medical advice to confirm the diagnosis of arthritis by using imaging and lab tests. Arthritis can be caused by a wide range of factors including inflammation as a result of wear and tear, infection, or a disease. Arthritis can affect various parts of the body including your joints, ankles, back, hands, and feet. You might experience arthritic pain continuously, acutely, or periodically.

Treatments that reduce and alleviate arthritis include physical therapy, medications, surgery, lifestyle changes, and home remedies. However, rather than using invasive procedures and commercial treatments, you can apply this healing salve three times a day to the part of the body you are experiencing pain. Note that care should be taken when using it to ensure that it does not come in contact with the mucosal tissue.

Since this healing salve uses cayenne essential oil, which can be an irritant to the eyes and mucosal tissue, be sure to wash your hands after applying it to your skin. Please note, the cayenne essential oil can also stain clothing and fabrics.

Ingredients
- One fl. oz. of Castor Oil (2 US Tbsps., 30ml)
- Eight fl. oz. of Coconut Oil, 100% Pure, Virgin, Unrefined (16 US Tbsp., 1 cup, 236ml)
- Four fl. oz. of Extra Virgin Olive Oil (8 US Tbsp., ½ cup, 118ml)
- 1000 IU of squeezed Vitamin E Oil from a capsule (optional)
- 50 drops of Cayenne Essential Oil

- 50 drops of Ginger Root Essential

Directions

1. Soften the coconut oil if necessary by placing the coconut oil container in a bowl of hot water. The water level should be no higher than half the container with the coconut oil.
2. Measure out the required amount of coconut oil into your 16 oz — Mason jar.
3. Next, add the essential oils and Vitamin E Oil to the coconut oil in the 16 oz. Mason jar.
4. Stir the oils into the coconut oil with stir sticks, stainless steel or wooden spoon.
5. Label your salve with the key essential oils, one use for the salve, and the date you made the salve.
6. Put a lid on the Mason jar and store at a temperature below 76 degrees (24 Celsius) to solidify.

Healing Salve for Nasal Congestion

Nasal congestion has a wide variety of causes and can result from any irritation to the nasal passages. These irritations could be an infection, an allergy, or tobacco smoke. Nasal congestion, informally called a "stuffy nose," may feel like pressure and the inability to breathe through the nostrils without difficulty.

Many people treat nasal congestion with over the counter medications such as a decongestant. Other solutions for nasal congestion include a Net pot, a nasal spray, or a humidifier. Be aware that this healing salve includes lemon essential oil which can create sensitivity to light. For that reason, do not apply this healing salve before exposure to the sun. If you expect to be exposed to the sun when this healing salve is needed, you may eliminate the lemon essential oil from the recipe, if helpful.

You can apply this healing salve to the top of the nose directly, or on the chest to inhale the vapors. If you decide to apply this salve to your nose, apply a small amount, enough to create a thin layer to avoid pore-clogging. Never apply any salve inside the nose or on the delicate mucosal tissue. Depending on the severity of the nasal congestion, you may apply this salve three times during 24 hours.

Ingredients

- One fl. oz. of Castor Oil (2 US Tbsp., 30ml)
- Eight fl. oz. of Coconut Oil, 100% Pure, Virgin, Unrefined (16 US Tbsp., 1 cup, 240ml)
- Four fl. oz. of Extra Virgin Olive Oil (8 US Tbsp., ½ cup, 120ml)
- 1000 IU of squeezed Vitamin E Oil from a capsule (optional)
- Twenty-five drops each of Eucalyptus to loosens mucus and treats respiratory inflammation, Lemon Essential Oil to boost the immune system, Peppermint Essential Oil to relieve pain, Rosemary Essential Oil to treat cough and sinus congestion and Thyme Essential Oil for antibacterial properties that treat respiratory infections.

Directions

1. Soften the coconut oil if necessary by placing the coconut oil container in a bowl of hot water. The water level should be no higher than half the container with the coconut oil.
2. Measure out the required amount of coconut oil into your 16 oz — Mason jar.
3. Next, add the essential oils, any other carrier oils, and Vitamin E Oil to the coconut oil in the 16 oz. Mason jar.
4. Stir the oils into the coconut oil with stir sticks, stainless steel or wooden spoon.
5. Label your salve with the key essential oils, one use for the salve, and the date you made the salve.
6. Put a lid on the Mason jar and store at a temperature below 76 degrees (24 Celsius) to solidify.

Healing Salve for Insomnia

Insomnia is the inability to fall asleep or stay asleep. Insomnia can be momentary, episodic, or enduring. You may experience insomnia due to stress, anxiety, your sleeping habits, a lack of exercise, a medical condition, or even as a side effect of medications.

Sleeping well is an important part of overall physical and emotional well-being. A lack of sleep, or poor sleep, can create numerous adverse effects on the mind, body, and even personal safety. This could include headaches, hallucinations, depression, irritability, poor coordination, or an inability to concentrate. A lack of sleep can also affect your immune system and the body's ability to repair and heal itself.

This healing salve includes essential oils with demonstrated abilities to relax the mind and reduce anxiety. If you are taking medications for insomnia or another condition, please consult a medical professional before applying this healing salve. You may apply this healing salve to your temples, your neck area, and your feet just before bedtime. After you apply this healing salve, be sure to deeply inhale and audibly exhale as you close your eyes to sleep.

Ingredients

- One fl. oz. of Castor Oil (2 US Tbsp. or 30ml)
- Eight fl. oz. of Coconut Oil, 100% Pure, Virgin, Unrefined (16 US Tbsp., 1 cup, or 236ml)
- Four fl. oz. of Extra Virgin Olive Oil (8 US Tbsp., ½ cup, or 120ml)
- 1000 IU of squeezed Vitamin E Oil from a capsule (this is optional)
- 50 drops of Chamomile Essential Oil for treatment of anxiety
- 50 drops of Lavender Essential Oil to induce relaxation

Direction

1. Soften the coconut oil if necessary by placing the coconut oil container in a bowl of hot water. The water level should be no higher than half the container with the coconut oil.

2. Measure out the required amount of coconut oil into your 16 oz — Mason jar.
3. Next, add the essential oils, any other carrier oils, and Vitamin E Oil to the coconut oil in the 16 oz. Mason jar.
4. Stir the oils into the coconut oil with stir sticks, stainless steel or wooden spoon.
5. Label your salve with the key essential oils, uses for the salve, and the date you made the salve.
6. Put a lid on the Mason jar and store at a temperature below 76 degrees (24 Celsius) to solidify.

Conclusion

From this book, we have learned so much about the natural ingredients that you can use to prepare homemade beauty, health, and home products. One thing that you have to bear in mind is that in this lifetime, we only have one body. In other words, your body has no spare part. That said, it is essential that we ensure that the products that we use daily maintain the natural glow of our skin and the overall health and beauty of our bodies. Whether the products that you use are applied directly onto your skin, ingested orally for your gut health or used around the home for cleaning, safety comes first!

The skin is one of the largest organs of the body and is considered one of the hardest working organs. It is the organ that protects you from exposure to harmful elements from our surrounding while ensuring that it regulates what the body takes in. So much of the aerosols in the environment contains particle contaminants that we cannot see, but the skin plays a central role in helping us filter them. Considering this heavy task that the skin does, it is necessary that you offer your body the right diet, sleep, water, and topical products that will maintain its natural glow.

Body scrubs, cleaning agents that we hold with our hands and the lotions/creams we apply directly to the skin are important to consider when we aim at maintaining a plump, soft baby skin. All these natural products that we have discussed ensure that our skin maintains its natural moisture while boosting skin rejuvenation by promoting skin cell regeneration. This is what gives you that healthy, youthful skin glow that will turn heads wherever you go. Ensure that every product that you use promotes moisture retention on your skin by simply serving as a shield against dehydration.

The ease of making all these DIY natural products for beauty, health, and home will make you an absolute believer in natural homemade products. Apart from the fact that these products are easy to make, they are clean, natural and pocket-friendly. It will simply make you feel good knowing that you are using clean products on your body and your home. Trust me; your skin will thank you for it.

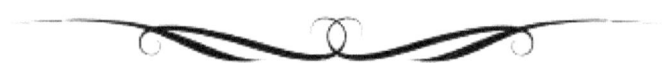

www.ingramcontent.com/pod-product-compliance
Lightning Source LLC
Chambersburg PA
CBHW050751290526
45792CB00008B/2142